Healthy Living Weight Loss Success Guide

Learn how to have proper nutrition and

weight management

Copyright Notice

Table of Contents

Forward

My experience with thousands of patients over the past 20+ years has taught me that a one-size weight-loss plan does not fit all. Individualized approaches to getting into shape work best–approaches in which people use programs customized to their own shapes and body composition, approaches that fit their lifestyles and their personalities.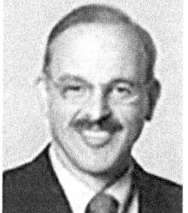

This success guide along with the help you can receive will help you to determine your plan needs. You will eat an amount of protein in your diet that is matched to the protein needs of your body, which will help you build or maintain lean muscle, which burns calories and which helps keep your metabolic rate up. You will learn how many calories you burn at rest and how fast you can lose weight on the number of calories in your personalized weight management Program. You will also learn what your target weight (based on the proper ratio of fat to lean) should be and see how it compares to what you think you should weigh.

If you tried to get all the protein you needed from foods such as meats, you would consume too many calories, because protein usually comes with extra fat calories in these foods. But by using a variety of Herbalife's delicious, protein-enriched, meal-replacement shakes, you can easily obtain the protein your body requires to build or maintain lean muscle mass and to feel full and satisfied. Herbalife's shakes, along with healthy meals, can help you realize easy and lasting weight loss. A healthy meal also is rich in colorful fruits and vegetables.

This is because the substances that give fruits and vegetables their "color" (called phytonutrients) can help prevent heart disease, common forms of cancer, some cases of nutrient-related and age-related blindness and more.

Your program guide also discusses the role of exercise in building lean body mass (muscle) and in reducing stress.

This plan is modeled on programs I use in my practice at the UCLA Center for Human Nutrition. For over 20 years, I have helped people learn about their individual bodies and, based on that, how to eat better and lose weight. Today, I am proud to be the chairman of the Scientific Advisory Board for Herbalife International, one of the largest distributors of high-quality meal replacements in the world. Herbalife has embraced the ideas and the science that I have used and proven in my practice. Through their worldwide network, they have provided me with the resources to finally be able to realize my dream of extending what I do in the office to millions of people worldwide. I hope this program helps you achieve your goals and your ideal weight.

David Heber, M.D., Ph.D.F.A.C.P., F.A.C.N., Professor of Medicine and Director, UCLA Center for Human Nutrition.

Introduction

In this we will try and show you aspects to proper eating and how to lose your excess weight in a healthy manner. We believe good nutrition leads to proper weight management.

First you need to understand how weight loss works:

If you eat the same number of calories as you burn, your weight remains the same.

If you eat fewer calories than you burn, you lose weight.

Your lean body mass which is everything in your body less the fat burns 14 calories per pound per day. More muscle means more calories are burnt doing the same thing.

To lose one pound per week, each day you must consume 500 fewer calories that your body burns.

With our quality products and proper exercise, you should lose 1-3 pounds per week in a healthy manner. The products that we use in Healthy Living is Herbalife.

Quality products...

We use only the highest research, development and manufacturing standards, including the finest raw ingredients, precise formulation and labeling, and trusted contract manufactures.

...Backed by acclaimed scientific leadership

Our renowned nutrition and scientific advisors partner in developing and testing products, using only the highest-quality ingredients and participating in sponsored, innovative university research worldwide.

We know that weight loss will take some time. Because of that we offer you a 15% discount through our site for our automatic renewal program. Just go to our site at http://herbalnutrition.com/rodstone, fill out the information form, contact us and we will establish you with an invoice to get you going on the road to success.

Rod

Understand Your Body – Your Personal Vision of Success

As you begin your personalized Healthy Weight Loss program, you need to understand your BMI. BMI is a reliable indicator of body fatness for most people. If your BMI score falls between 18.5 to 24.9, you are in a healthy weight range. In such case, you may still push through with the healthy weight loss program as Herbalife products do not only let you lose weight, but also regulate and maintain the right amount of nutrients to your body, letting you achieve a better weight and healthier lifestyle. Following the program, you will also notice the shaping effects Herbalife products have on your body and slowly getting the curve that you have always wanted.

This chart provides you with what is determined to be underweight, normal, overweight or obesity in reference to BMI:

	BMI
Underweight	Below 18.5
Normal	18.5 – 24.9
Overweight	25.0 – 29.9
Obesity	30.0 and Above

You can find your actual BMI by checking it out at our site at: http://herbalnutrition.com/resources/showbmicalculator/distributor/rodstone

This will show you some of the ideal weights based on frame size:

WOMEN				MEN			
Height Ft. In.	Frame Size			Height Ft. In.	Frame Size		
	Small	Med.	Large		Small	Med.	Large
4'10"	102-111	109-121	118-131	5'2"	128-134	131-141	138-150
4'11"	103-113	111-123	120-134	5'3"	130-136	133-143	140-153
5'0"	104-115	113-126	122-137	5'4"	132-138	135-145	142-156
5'1"	106-118	115-129	125-140	5'5"	134-140	137-148	144-160
5'2"	108-121	118-132	128-143	5'6"	136-142	139-151	146-164
5'3"	111-124	121-135	131-147	5'7"	138-145	142-154	149-168
5'4"	114-127	124-138	134-151	5'8"	140-148	145-157	152-172
5'5"	117-130	127-141	137-155	5'9"	142-151	156-160	155-176
5'6"	120-133	130-144	140-159	5'10"	144-154	151-163	158-180
5'7"	123-136	133-144	143-163	5'11"	146-157	154-166	161-184
5'8"	126-139	136-150	146-167	6'0"	149-160	157-170	164-188
5'9"	129-142	139-153	149-170	6'1"	152-164	160-174	168-192
5'10"	132-145	142-156	152-173	6'2"	155-168	165-178	172-197
5'11"	135-148	145-159	155-176	6'3"	158-172	167-182	176-202
6'0"	138-151	148-162	158-176	6'4"	162-176	171-187	181-207

Calories are what people seem to look at when they are determining dieting. Calories are units of energy your body uses to fuel its functions and activities created from protein, fats and carbohydrates found in our foods and beverages necessary for basic body functions like keeping your body functioning.

The number of calories we need each day depends on how much we should weight, how much muscle mass we have and how active we are.

A pound = approximately 3,500 calories.

- A gram of protein = 4 calories
- A gram of Carbohydrate = 4 calories
- A gram of fat = 9 calories

A woman needs 12 calories for every pound of body weight and a man needs 14 calories for every pound of body weight.

The chart below gives you daily calorie needs by weight:

Women lbs	Calories	Men lbs
100	1200	
125	1500	107
150	1800	129
167	2000	143

	2400	171
	2700	193

A major thing to remember with your weight loss is that it took time for the extra weight to get on your body. It will take some time in order for you to reach your healthy goal. With the Basic Healthy Weight Loss program you can figure on 1-2 pounds of weight loss per week. And with the Ultimate Healthy Weight Loss program you can figure on 2-4 pounds of weight loss per week.

As you begin your Healthy Weight Loss program, look ahead toward your destination. Write down your goals and paste a current photo of yourself below. When you've reached your weight goal, add a photo of the new you. You'll be amazed at the difference.

The Starting You

The New You

Current Weight:	Current Weight:
Target Weight:	
Current Waist:	Current Waist:
Target Waist:	
Current Neck:	Current Neck:
Target Waist:	
Current Chest:	Current Chest:
Target Chest:	
Current Arms:	Current Arms:

Target Arms:	
Current Hips:	Current Hips:
Target Hips:	
Current Thighs:	Current Thighs:
Target Thighs:	
Current Calves:	Current Calves:
Target Calves:	

My reason for wanting to lose weight:

1.

2.

3.

What Shape are you?

Shape and weight are related, but they're not the same thing. You have inherited one of the natural body shapes, often referred to as apple shape and pear shape.

Find the shape closest to yours on the charts below.

Circle the shape you are and the shape you want to be.

No matter what your shape is, your goal is to move your shape toward the left on the chart, by reducing fat and increasing your lean body mass.

Female-Pear

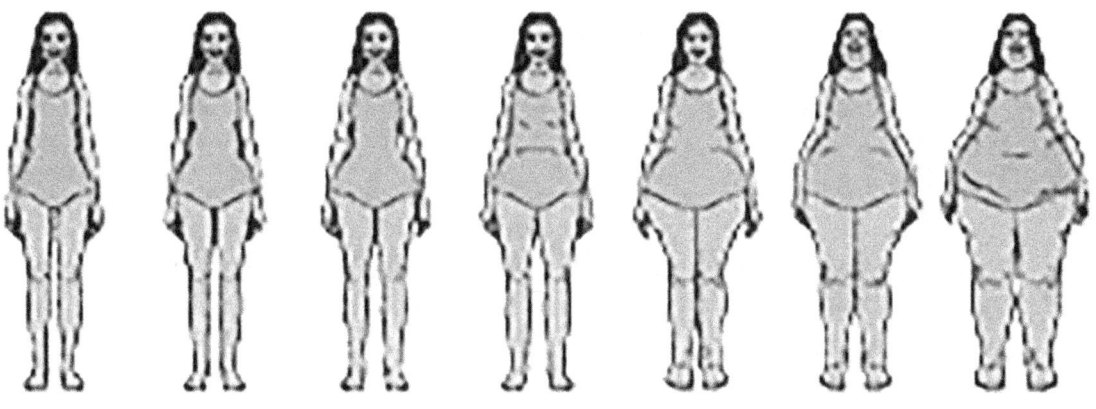

Female-Apple

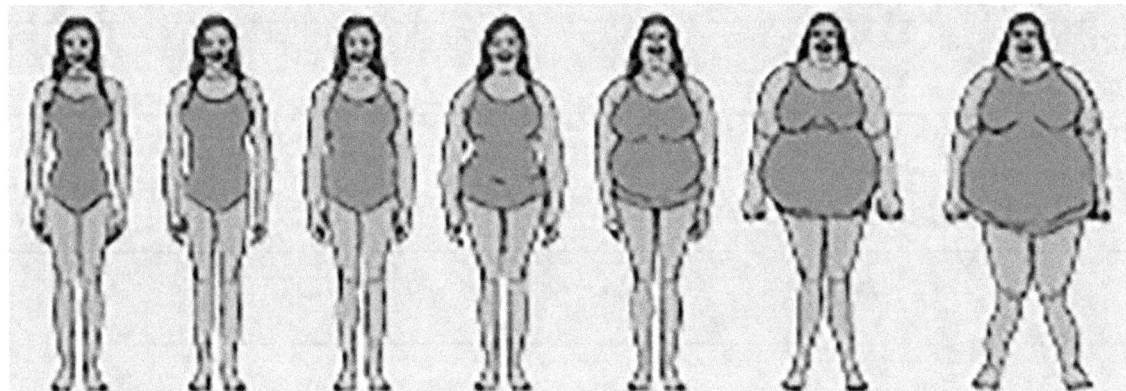

Male-Apple

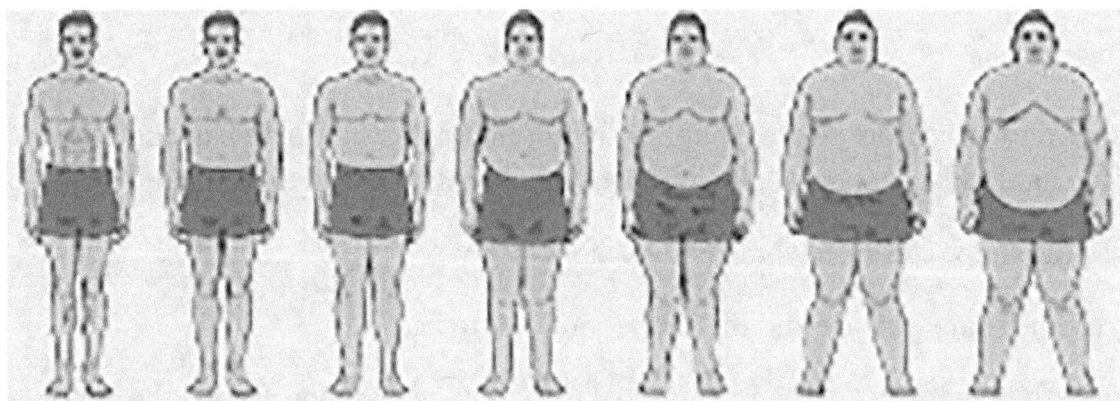

What Your Shape means

If you are Apple-Shaped

You carry fat in your upper body; face, neck, chest and waist. Many women and almost all men are apple-shaped.

- Upper-body fat is usually caused by diet and lack of exercise.
- Fat around the waist usually means that there is also internal fat, which may cause serious health problems.
- Reducing internal fat can dramatically improve your health.
- Cutting calories alone will not eliminate upper body fat.

- To lose this weight, remodel your lean fat body mass ratio with the Herbalife Healthy Meal program of meal management, protein and exercise.

If you are Pear-Shaped

You carry fat in your lower body: hips and thighs.

Pear-shaped people are predominately women.

- Lower-body fat is partially inherited, partially a result of diet.
- This type of fat does not cause specific health problems.
- Cutting calories and increasing exercise may not be sufficient to reduce lower body fat.
- Eating more protein along with specific lower-body workout routines can tone and improve lower body shape.

Whatever shape you're in, the Healthy Living Herbalife program can help you improve your shape, health and your life!

It's not just your weight, it's your body composition.

Healthy target weight is based on your body type and your ratio of lean body mass to body fat. Lean body mass includes your muscles, bone, minerals and other nonfat tissue in your body. The more muscle mass you have, the more calories your body burns.

Remember, you need a certain amount of body fat for good health. It stores the energy your muscles need and serves as your body's shock absorber. Too little body fat can be as unhealthy as too much.

The National Institutes of Health warns that excess body fat frequently results in significant impairment of health. The chart below shows estimated target-fat percentages for men and women at different ages.

Men		Women	
Age	Target body fat	Age	Target body fat
19-39	11% - 16%	19-39	19% - 21%
40-50+	17.5% - 20%	40-50+	22.5% - 25%

You need protein to stay strong and healthy. If you don't eat enough of it every day, your body will steal protein from your muscles and organs.

The general daily dietary guidelines are:

- protein –15% - 25%
- carbohydrates – 55% - 75%
- fat – 10% - 20%

Protein 101

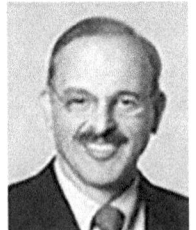

By David Heber, M.D., Ph.D. Director the UCLA Center for Human Nutrition

It seems everywhere we look, someone is promoting a new diet that praises the power of protein. But whether you want to lose, gain, or maintain your current weight, the importance of protein goes far beyond physical appearance and muscle building.

A necessity for every body

Protein is an important component of every cell in the body. It is an organic compound, composed of 22 amino acids, otherwise known as the building blocks of life. Protein is stored in muscles and organs and the body utilizes it to build and repair tissues, as well as for the production of enzymes and hormones. Proteins also make it possible for blood to carry oxygen throughout the body. Along with fat and carbohydrates, protein is a "macronutrient," meaning the body needs relatively large amounts of it. The Institute of Medicine of the National Academy of Sciences has concluded that our daily protein requirements should be 10% to 35% of our total caloric intake, with men needing slightly more than women. A lack of protein can cause loss of muscle mass, decreased immunity, as well as weakening of the heart and respiratory system.

Recent studies recommend eating one gram of protein per pound of lean body mass each day. This is more protein than former guidelines: an average of 100 grams per day for women and 150 grams per day for men. People's protein needs must be calculated using their individual body types and lean body mass.

How protein affects your weight

The widespread popularity of high-protein diets is due in large part to their ability to help manage hunger. When protein is absorbed, it sends a signal to the brain to decrease your hunger. Another benefit of protein is that it raises your resting metabolism by maintaining muscle mass. As we age, muscle mass decreases without exercise, so staying fit is a key to burning fat by keeping your metabolism high. Protein also leads to a much less rapid rise and fall of blood sugar and insulin, so you avoid the "sugar highs and lows" after eating sweets without adequate protein. Certain foods, however, provide a healthier resource for protein than others.

Consider the source

You can obtain healthy sources of protein without high levels of saturated fat. For example, soybeans, nuts and whole grains provide protein without much saturated fat and offer plenty of healthful fiber and micronutrients as well. If you're looking for yet another great way to obtain healthy protein, vegetable sources of protein found in Herbalife's Formula 1, are high-quality and have lower calorie levels with virtually no added fat. Herbalife® products personalize your daily protein intake to match your body's needs. With a variety of shakes and snacks, the Herbalife® program helps you build or maintain lean muscle while providing healthy weight management support.

Soy protein: is the highest quality plant protein available. It's an excellent source for the amino acids your body needs, as well as antioxidants to help you maintain healthy cells.

Whey protein: provides more amino acids and mixes well with nonfat (skim) milk or soy milk to create creamy, delicious shakes.

Now that you've increased your knowledge of protein, you can effectively enhance your diet and allow good health to take shape.

The proper mix of protein and carbohydrates will provide you with energy for longer periods of time than some types. Check out this chart:

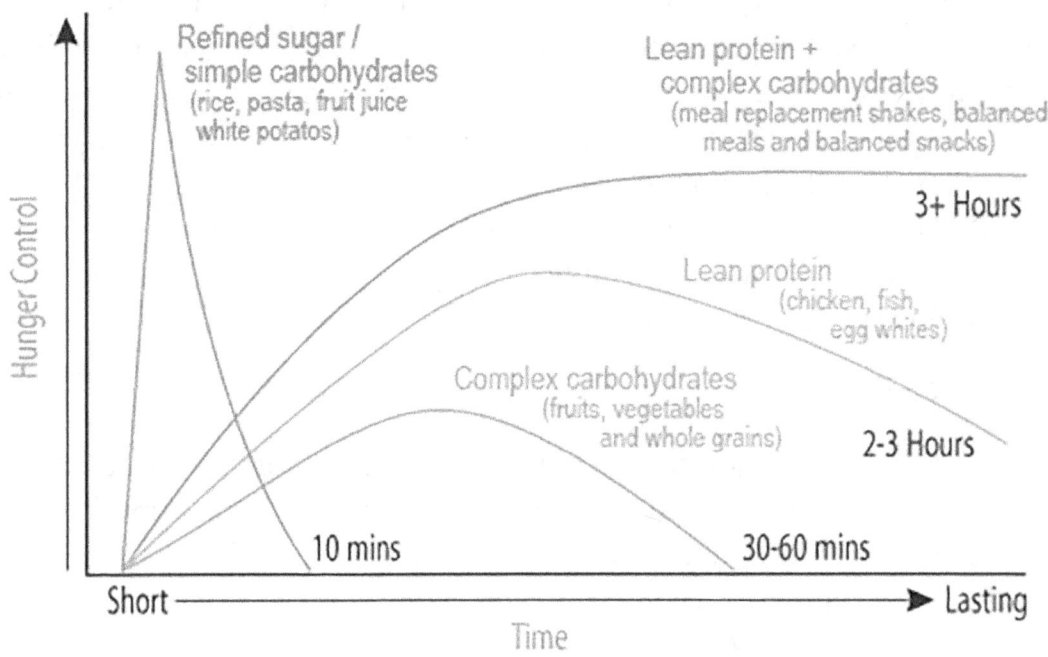

Your Plan Makes It Work

So you need to get enough protein as you control your calories. How does that work in the real world? Look at the chart below. See how Herbalife Meal replacement, snacks and a balanced daily meal make your program work for you!

Meal Planning Chart								
Daily calories	1,200		1,500		1,800		2,400	
Daily protein								
Breakfast	Protein	Calories	Protein	Calories	Protein	Calories	Protein	Calories
*Formula 1 shake								
*Milk type (8 oz)								
*1 portion fruit								
*Protein powder								
supplements								

snack	Protein	Calories	Protein	Calories	Protein	Calories	Protein	Calories
**Protein rich								
lunch	Protein	Calories	Protein	Calories	Protein	Calories	Protein	Calories
*Formula 1 shake								
*Milk type (8 oz)								
*1 portion fruit								
Protein powder								
supplements								
snack	Protein	Calories	Protein	Calories	Protein	Calories	Protein	Calories
**Protein rich								
Colorful Dinner	Protein	Calories	Protein	Calories	Protein	Calories	Protein	Calories
Protein								
Vegetable								
Fruit								
supplements								
Daily protein & calorie totals								

*Formula 1 shake is 2 T Formula 1, 8 oz. milk type, 1 portion fruit, personalized protein powder of 1-3 T based on needs for your body.

** Protein rich snacks should be 10-20 grams of protein and 60 – 160 calories.

Your milk type choice is whatever low fat soy, dairy, etc. that has at least 5 grams or more per 8 oz.

A 25-30 grams protein portion of lean meat is about the size of your palm or a deck of playing cards.

Carbohydrates

Carbohydrates are necessary to your health, because every cell in your body uses them for energy. In fact, your brain can only use carbohydrates for energy.

With the popularity of low-carb diets, many people are afraid to eat any carbohydrates, but it is important to distinguish between the health-robbing effects of simple sugars and other carbs, and the health-giving properties of complex carbohydrates.

Complex carbohydrates are high-fiber foods, which improve your digestion. They help stabilize the blood sugar, keep your energy at an even level, and help you feel satisfied longer after your meal.

In contrast, sugar and other simple carbohydrates can alter your mood, lead to cravings and compulsive eating, cause wide swings in your blood-sugar levels, and cause weight gain in most people. In addition, a high consumption of sugar can lead to uncomfortable withdrawal symptoms when you finally decide to improve your diet and forgo the sweets.

Some examples of healthy foods containing complex carbohydrates:

Spinach	Whole Barley	Grapefruit
Turnip Greens	Buckwheat	Apples
Lettuce	Buckwheat bread	Prunes
Water Cress	Oat bran bread	Apricots, Dried
Zucchini	Oatmeal	Pears
Asparagus	Oat bran cereal	Plums
Artichokes	Museli	Strawberries
Okra	Wild rice	Oranges
Cabbage	Brown rice	Yams
Celery	Multi-grain bread	Carrots
Cucumbers	Pinto beans	Potatoes
Dill Pickles	Yogurt, low fat	Soybeans
Radishes	Skim milk	Lentils
Broccoli	Navy beans	Garbanzo beans

Brussels Sprouts	Cauliflower	Kidney beans
Eggplant	Soy milk	Lentils
Onions	Whole meal spelt bread	Split peas

Some examples of foods containing simple carbohydrates:

Simple carbohydrates are more refined, are usually found in foods with fewer nutrients, and tend to be less satisfying and more fattening.

Table sugar

Corn syrup

Fruit juice

Candy

Cake

Bread made with white flour

Pasta made with white flour

Soda pop, such as Coke®, Pepsi®, Mountain Dew®, etc.

Candy

All baked goods made with white flour

Most packaged cereals

The closer you get to nature, the closer you get to health.

Simple carbohydrates, like sugar and corn syrup, are created in a factory – while complex carbohydrates in vegetables and whole grains are designed by nature, and help you maintain your health.

Why not brown and beige?

We all know that eating plenty of fruits and vegetables is the way to better health, but we often settle for food that is quick, easy and inexpensive. Many of these easy meals are brown or beige, filled with calories from added fat, sugar and starch: too many calories and too few healthful nutrients.

To build a healthy eating plan, always choose colors. Colorful fruits and vegetables are full of vitamins and minerals, and they provide omega-3 fatty acids. These "good" fats stimulate your immune system and sup- port your body's defense against infections and tumors. The more colorful your meal, the healthier it is. Tonight, make your dinner plate look lively! Fill two-thirds of it with colorful fruits and vegetables. Those colors mean good nutrition and lower calories, too.

Fruits and vegetables are the foundation of your daily menus. They help maintain your organs and immune system, keeping your body strong as the weight comes off.

Simply eating more fruits and vegetables is not the answer–they must be the right fruits and vegetables. Starchy vegetables such as peas or lentils (200 to 250 calories per cup) are healthy, but they contain more calories than you may want. If you need to eat more to satisfy your hunger, add low-calorie vegetables. For example, spinach and asparagus are better choices than higher-calorie corn and peas. A cup of spinach topped with a 2 cup of tomato sauce has only about 90 calories, but it gives you nutrients from two color groups.

Colorful foods provide nutrition from the family of chemicals called phytonutrients, or "plant" nutrients. These substances contribute to your healthy food program.

There are seven colors of fruits and vegetables that you should have daily.

Use the chart below to plan a colorful, delicious, personalized menu every day!

Color	Food item	Portion	Calories
Red Purple	Beets, cooked	1C	75
	Eggplant, cooked	1C	30
	Red cabbage, cooked	1C	30
	Blackberries	1C	75
	Blueberries	1C	110
	Grapes	1C	115
	Plums	2 small	70
	Prunes	3 whole	60
	Red apple	1 medium	100
	Red pear	1 medium	100
	Red wine	4 oz. glass	80
	Strawberries	1 C, sliced	50

	Peppers, red chopped	1 C	30
Red	Tomato juice	1 C	40
	Tomato sauce or puree	1 C	100
	Tomato soup, made with water	1 C	85
	Tomato vegetable juice	1 C	45
	Tomatoes, cooked	1 C	70
	Pink grapefruit	1 fruit	40
	Pink grapefruit juice	1 C	50
	Watermelon	1 C balls	50
	Tomatoes, raw, chopped	1 C	40
Orange	Acorn Squash, baked	1C	85
	Carrots, cooked	1C	70
	Pumpkin, cooked	1C	50
	Sweet Potato	1C	200
	Winter Squash, baked	1C	70
	Apricots	3 whole	50
	Cantaloupe	1C cubes	55
	Mango	1 large	80
	Carrots, raw	1C	50
Orange/Yellow	Nectarine	1 large	70
	Orange	1 large	85
	Orange Juice	1 C	50
	Papaya	1 large	75
	Peach	1 large	70
	Pineapple	1 C, diced	75
	Tangerine	1 medium	45
	Yellow Grapefruit	1 fruit	40
Yellow/Green	Collard Greens, cooked	1 C	50
	Corn	1 ear	75
	Green Beans, cooked	1 C	45

	Green Peas	1 C	140
	Mustard Greens, cooked	1 C	20
	Spinach, cooked	1 C	40
	Turnip Greens, cooked	1 C	30
	Zucchini, with skin, cooked	1 C	30
	Avocado	1 average fruit	80
	Honeydew	1 C cubes	60
	Kiwi	1 large	55
	Cucumber	1 C	15
	Pepper, green, chopped	1 C	30
	Pepper, yellow, chopped	1 C	30
	Romaine Lettuce	1 C	10
	Spinach, raw	1 C	10
Green	Broccoli, cooked	1 C	45
	Brussels Sprouts	1 C	60
	Cabbage, cooked	1 C	35
	Cauliflower, cooked	1 C	30
	Chinese Cabbage, cooked	1 C	20
	Kale, cooked	1 C	35
	Swiss Chard, cooked	1 C	20
	Cabbage, raw	1 C	20
White/Green	Artichoke	1 medium	60
	Asparagus	1 C	45
	Celery, diced	1 C	20
	Leeks, cooked	1 C	30
	Mushrooms, cooked	1 C	40
	Onion, cooked	1 C	105
	Endive, raw	1 C	10

Carbohydrates: Good News/Bad News

Your body converts carbohydrates into sugar, which gives you energy. That's the good news. The bad news is that some carbohydrate foods turn into too much sugar too fast, with too many calories. You can identify which carbohydrates are good for you and which to avoid by checking their glycemic index and glycemic load.

Glycemic Index measures how fast the carbohydrates in a food turn into sugar in the body. Foods with a high glycemic index convert into sugar very quickly, with negative physical effects. Foods with a low glycemic index turn into sugar gradually, helping maintain your body's chemical balance. In general, foods with a low index are preferable.

Glycemic Load measures the amount of sugar a food actually releases in the body. Foods with a low glycemic load usually have a low glycemic index. They are good choices for your meal plan. Foods with a high glycemic load can have from very low to very high indexes. You should avoid high load foods as a regular part of your meal plan.

When you choose carbohydrate foods, always check both their glycemic index and glycemic load. Detailed tables with this information are widely available. Use the chart below to get started.

High Glycemic Index		Medium Glycemic Index		Low Glycemic Index	
Fruits and Vegetables	Starches	Fruits and	Starches	Fruits and Vegetables	Starches
Banana*	Bagel	Apricot*	Oatmeal	Apple	Lentils
Raisins	Bread (whole	Cantalou	Kidney Beans*	Asparagus	
Beets*	grain)	pe	Pita Bread	Broccoli	
	Carrots*	Grapes*	Navy Beans	Brussel Sprouts	
	Cereals	Pineapple*	Yam/Sweet	Cauliflower	
	Corn	Watermelon	Potatoes	Celery	
	Granola Kidney			Cherries	
	Beans Muffin			Cucumber	
	(bran)			Grapefruit Green	
	Pasta			Beans Green	
	Potatoes			Pepper	
	Pretzels Refined			Kiwi	
	Sugar Rice			Lettuce	
				Mushrooms	
				Onions Orange	
				Peach	
	Tortilla (wheat)				
				Plums	
				Spinach	
				Strawberries	
				Tomatoes	
				Zucchini	

Fats Essentials

Fats are very confusing to most of us.

<u>Saturated Fats</u> basically come from animals and dairy. (Butter and Lard)

<u>Monounsaturated Fats</u> come from some vegetables, poultry and nuts. (Olives, Nuts, Poultry Fat, Avocadoes)

<u>Polyunsaturated Fats</u> include what we call essential fats, because they must be eaten and are essential to our health as well.

<u>Omega – 3</u> (DHA and EPA) come primarily from cold water fish that feed on plankton. It is also found in flax, fig and raspberry seeds.

<u>Omega – 6</u> comes from vegetable oils, grain, and arachadonic acid from egg yolks and red meat.

These essential polyunsaturated fats (Omega – 3 and Omega – 6) make the cells membrane flexible. This helps them to be more insulin sensitive. The Omega – 3 and Omega – 6 are transformed into Eicosanoids. Eicosanoids are the most biologically active of all substances in the body. They are required to work in concert in order to achieve fine control of various psychological and physiological processes.

Omega – 6
> - Causes the blood to be more prone to clot.
> - Promote rapid growth of cells.
> - Induce smooth muscles cells to contract.
> - Bring about an inflammatory response.
> - Cause pain.

Omega – 3
> - Blood Thinner
> - Slows the growth of cells
> - Relaxes smooth muscle contractions
> - Anti inflammatory response
> - Relieve Pain
> - Replaces and repairs the nerves and brain.

Improve your ratio

During ancient times when we were hunter/gather the ratio of Omega 6 to Omega 3 was 2:1.

The typical American Diet today is 20-50:1.

The Omega – 6 are the ones that cause pain, inflammation, smooth muscle contractions, blood clotting, etc. The Omega – 6 are found primarily in seeds, which means grain and grain products.

<u>Increased levels of Omega 6 in the diet is directly linked to increased heart disease, insulin resistance, cancer, diabetes, neurological diseases, and accelerated aging.</u>

Today we also eat a new kind of fat that is totally artificial. These are usually identified as "Partially Hydrogenated Oil." They have a long shelf life. They are stable. They are sold in a clear glass bottle. They make lots of money for the manufactures. They are <u>deadly</u>. These are the trans fats and many have been removed. But they are still around and you need to be careful.

We moved from butter to margarine. We moved from lard to corn oil and safflower oil Here is known problems with these fats:

- Lower HDL (good cholesterol)
- Raise LDL (bad cholesterol)
- Decrease Testosterone
- Increase production of abnormal sperm
- Decrease amount of cream in breast milk
- Weaken the immune response
- Increase the production of free radicals
- Decrease response of insulin receptors
- Causes hyperinsulinemia

You find the highest levels of trans fats in bakery goods, in sandwich cookies, in vanilla wafers, in animal crackers, and in honey graham crackers. This is what we are feeding our children's brains.

The following diseases have been associated with fat problems in the brain:

- Depression
- Memory loss
- Violence
- Bi-polar disease
- Schizophrenia
- Alzheimer's
- Multiple Sclerosis
- Parkinson's Disease
- ADD and ADHD
- Learning Disabilities
- Behavior Problems

You need to use no trans fats, use a pharmaceutical grade fish oil daily, decrease Omega 6 by limiting grain, use olive oil whenever possible for cooking and salads.

Pharmaceutical grade fish oil is not the kind you buy at a vitamin store of discount store or corner drug store. It is approximately $25 for a bottle of 100. It takes approximately 100 gallons of health food store cheap fish oil to make 1 gallon of pharmaceutical grade fish oil.

How to Understand Food Labels - How To Read Food Labels

When trying to figure out what the food you are thinking of buying actually contains, ignore the front of the package hype! It is just that - marketing hype. Manufacturers can't actually lie on labeling, but they can stretch the true when trying to get your attention to buy their product.

Every packaged food must include a list of ingredients. The ingredient in largest quantity is listed first, while the one in smallest quantity is listed last.

Nutrition Facts

Serving Size 4 oz. (113g)
Servings Per Container 4

Amount Per Serving

Calories 280   Calories from Fat 130

	% Daily Value*
Total Fat 14g	22%
Saturated Fat 3.5g	18%
Trans Fat 2.5g	
Cholesterol 120mg	40%
Sodium 640mg	27%
Total Carbohydrate 13g	4%
Dietary Fiber 1g	4%
Sugars 0g	
Protein 24g	

Vitamin A 2%	•	Vitamin C 2%
Calcium 2%	•	Iron 6%

*Percent Daily Values are based on a 2,000 calorie diet. Your daily values may be higher or lower depending on your calorie needs:

		Calories	2,000	2,500
Total Fat	Less Than		65g	80g
Saturated Fat	Less Than		20g	25g
Cholesterol	Less Than		300mg	300 mg
Sodium	Less Than		2,400mg	2,400mg
Total Carbohydrate			300g	375g
Dietary Fiber			25g	30g

Calories per gram:
Fat 9 • Carbohydrate 4 • Protein 4

Recommended serving size/Calories per serving. The first items, at the top of the label, you'll notice are Serving Size and Servings Per Container. Serving Size is a standard measure of food. Servings Per Container represents the number of servings found in the food package. Serving size can be expressed in kitchen terms - cups, spoons, slices, ounces, and also in grams. Serving size tells how much food makes up a single serving. All data on the label is based on the serving size stated.

Amount Per Serving - Shows the number of calories found in a single food serving. Multiply this number by the serving size and it should equal, or come close to, the total volume of the package.

Calories from fat - Food labels show Calories from Fat so you can limit the amount of fat you eat for a healthier diet. The rule of thumb is that no more than 30% of your daily calories should come from fat. Higher fat foods should be eaten in smaller portions.

% Daily Value - This section tells you what percentage of the total recommended daily amount of each nutrient (fats, carbs, proteins, major vitamins, and minerals) is in each serving, based on a 2,000 calorie per day diet.

Total Fat - This equals the number of grams of fat per serving of the food. A heart-healthy diet limits foods containing saturated fats, trans fats, cholesterol, and sodium.

Saturated Fat - A fat that is solid at room temperature and comes chiefly from animal food products and some plants. Some examples of saturated fat include foods such as beef, lamb, pork, lard, butter, cream, whole milk and high fat cheese. Plant sources include coconut oil, cocoa butter, palm oil and palm kernel oil. Saturated fat causes high LDL cholesterol levels -- a risk for cardiovascular disease.

Trans Fat - Also known as also known as trans fatty acid. Trans fat is a specific type of fat formed when liquid fats are made into solid fats by the addition of hydrogen atoms, in a process strangely enough known as hydrogenation. Hydrogenation solidifies liquid oils and increases the shelf life and the flavor stability of oils and foods that contain them. Trans fat is found in vegetable shortenings and in some margarines, crackers, cookies, snack foods and other foods. Small amounts of trans fats are found naturally in certain animal based foods. Trans fat is what is considered unhealthy fat.

Cholesterol - This line tells you how many milligrams of cholesterol and what percent this is of the recommended daily value.

Sodium/salt - The latest recommendation for sodium is less than 2,400 mg of sodium per day, or about a teaspoon of table salt.

Total carbohydrates - Tells you how many grams of carbohydrates are in each serving and the percentage of the Daily Value this represents. This number includes starches, complex carbohydrates, dietary fiber, added sugar sweeteners, and non-digestible additives.

Fiber - Fiber is an indigestible carbohydrate and aids in elimination. At least 15 grams of fiber per day is recommended.

Protein - Many foods contain some protein but meat, fish, poultry and dairy foods are highest. Protein needs average between 50-100 grams per day.

Percent Daily Values - This section gives some estimated nutrients per 2000 and 2500 calories.

Proper Digestion Can Help Weight Loss

It has been said, that poor digestion is synonym with poor nutrition. You might be getting the proper nutrients into your body, but your system isn't able to absorb it. Proper digestive functioning is needed to reduce hunger, to gain the nutrients you need, and to offer you proper energy levels for effective weight management.

It is difficult to lose weight if you have poor digestion. Improper digestion is usually the cause of most weight problems.

Poor digestion takes a lot out of your body, and makes it weak, leaving it more vulnerable to attacks from other sources. If your digestive processes are not functioning at their peak, you may feel tired, weak, exhausted, constantly hungry and dissatisfied. Improper digestion can also affect your mood and your overall health; so, to lose weight, you should optimize your digestive processes.

Proteins and Digestion

In "Eat Carbs, Lose Weight: Drop All the Pounds You Want without Giving Up the Foods You Love," authors Denise Austin and Amy Campbell M.S. R.D. C.D.E. explain how digestive processes aid weight loss practices. In discussing protein consumption, the authors explain that consuming proteins helps to slow down digestive processes, which in turn, slows down the entry of sugars into your bloodstream. When this happens, you develop a sensation of being full faster. When you feel full, you will cease eating and will consume fewer calories; this will help you reduce your overall caloric intake, so you can lose weight more readily.

Carbohydrates and Digestion

Austin and Campbell argue that you should also break up your carbohydrate consumption throughout the day and eat smaller meals to help you stabilize your blood sugar levels. A drop in blood sugar levels could make you feel hungry when you really are not. Further, since you will be breaking your meals up into smaller portions, your digestive system will be working more frequently throughout the day to digest foods; this will also improve your sense of being full and diminish your hunger cravings.

The Effects of Rapid Eating and Stress

In "Eat More, Weigh Less: Dr. Dean Ornish's Program for Losing Weight Safely While Eating Abundantly," Dr. Dean Ornish explains that stressful emotions and rapid eating have an effect on your digestive processes that may actually cause you to gain weight. Since the act of eating involves satiating your hunger, eating too fast can cause you to fail to get any enjoyment out of the foods you consume; this may cause you to eat more and to gain weight.

In addition, Dr. Ornish writes that during stressful periods, your digestion is negatively affected; your body will shunt blood away from the digestive system when you are stressed. When you are not getting enough blood and energy to your digestive system, your body will fail to absorb the nutrients it needs from the foods you consume. Finally, Dr. Ornish says that whenever you are emotionally stressed your mouth will reduce its production of saliva and the alpha-amylase enzyme: an enzyme needed for the first stage of digestion. The latter will reduce proper nutrient absorption as well.

Malabsorption

If your digestive system is not working properly, there is a possibility that you will not get all of the nutrients you can from the foods you consume. In "Nutritional Biochemistry," Tom Brody explains that a lack of nutrients and issues with malabsorption can develop into health conditions, such as anemia, that can make you feel tired and fatigued. These conditions will do little for your energy levels and you will have less motivation to exercise and lose weight.

Improve Digestion

Digestion of food is the most energy consuming thing your body does. It's the same reason you hear your mom say "wait one hour after eating before swimming". It's not because you'll get cramps, it's because your body has sent so much blood to your stomach to do the work of digestion that you will have less energy for swimming.

Let me ask you this: If you don't get the nutrition out of the food you're eating, why are you eating it? That's the whole point isn't it? Making a few simple changes to how you eat, you can then assimilate all the nutrients, vitamins, minerals, fats, enzymes and protein of which your body is built.

Chew Each Bite Of Food At Least 30 Times

Digestion starts in the mouth. It's where the breakdown of the food first occurs. Our saliva mixes with our food during the chewing process, but only if you keep it in your mouth for awhile. If you make an effort to slow down and chew each bite of food at least 30 times, you not only take a great deal of effort off the stomach in breaking down the food, you also mix the food with your saliva, further enhancing the digestion process.

Remember, digestion of food is the most energy consuming thing your body does. Help out your stomach by chewing your food, turning it into a mush with your teeth and mixing it with your saliva. Improve your digestion, release more energy, get more nutrition out of your food and you may find that you drop a few pounds and feel better. Do this for 21 days, anchor the habit and record your results.

Eat Your Meal Slowly

By simply slowing down, your stomach has time to tell your brain that it's full. You don't have to finish all the food on your plate either. When you're full, you're full.

Never Eat To Capacity

Have you ever seen a picture of your stomach? Your stomach is a muscle that churns your food along with the digestive juices it cranks out. Your stomach needs room for this churning to take place and if it's full to capacity, proper digestion won't take place. Remember, digestion is very energy consuming. The energy you save could better be put to cleaning your body, burning fat or for workouts at the gym.

Think of your stomach in thirds. One third food, one third liquid and one third empty for the digestion process. You'll be much better off, be able to digest your food completely and get full nutritional value from it if it's completely digested.

Eat More Fiber

A majority of Americans consume only about 14 grams of fiber per day. The Institute of Medicine recommends 38 grams for men and 25 grams for women. Studies around the world find that people who eat 40-60 grams of fiber a day have the least body fat.

In his book, "Health Secrets of the Stone Age," Dr Philip Goscienski, M.D., stated that they ate 60-150 grams per day. Some of the other interesting comparisons are:

	Stone Age	Contemporary American
Dietary protein	33 %	12 %
Carbohydrate	46 %	46 %
Fat	21%	42%
Fiber	60-150 grams	10-20 grams

Sodium	700 milligrams	2300-6900 milligrams
Calcium	1500-2000 milligrams	740 milligrams
Sugar	Rare	1/3 lb./day
Vitamin C	440 milligrams	88 milligrams
Alcohol	None	7-10% of daily calories

How Weight Loss Works

If you eat the same number of calories as you burn, your weight remains the same.

Energy in   Energy Out

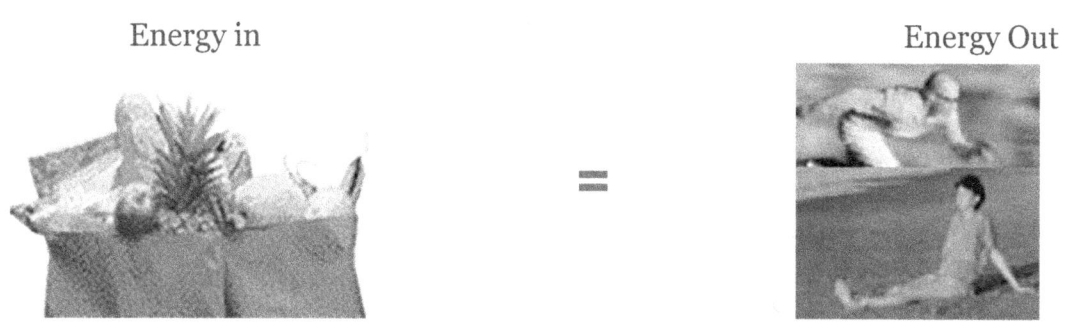

If you eat fewer calories than you burn, you lose weight.

Energy in   Energy Out

Your lean body mass which is everything in your body less the fat burns 14 calories per pound per day. More muscle means more calories are burnt doing the same thing.

To lose one pound per week, each day you must consume 500 fewer calories that your body burns.

This is why the "fast weight loss" that you see promised is not within the healthy guidelines of how your body works.

This is why we offer you the automatic program:

- Go to our site http://herbalnutrition.com/rodstone
- Fill out your information
- Send us a mailing through contact us
- We will establish you an invoice so we can provide you with your monthly requirements
- We will automatically charge your card and send you your products at 15% off the regular price.
- You can stop or make changes any time.

Trigger Foods

Trigger Foods are the ones that you love and crave. They make you feel good while you eat them. Then, they make you feel guilty because you know they're putting on the pounds. Have you ever started with just one potato chip or one chocolate-chip cookie and ended up eating the whole bag? Those little snacks can add up to big doses of fat and calories.

Which of these sweet, creamy or salty snacks do you crave?

- Chips, peanuts, crackers, pretzels
- Cheese, pizza
- Mayonnaise, margarine, butter
- Red meat, fatty fish
- Cola, juice
- Cakes, pastries, cookies, muffins
- Ice cream, frozen yogurt
- Chocolate

Look at the damage that Trigger Foods can do to your meal plan:

- Peanuts (1 cup) 835 calories, 71 grams of fat
- Corn chips (7 oz) 1,065 calories, 66 grams of fat
- Chocolate-chip cookies (6 small) 350 calories, 16 grams of fat
- Bagel and cream cheese (1 bagel 2 tsp cream cheese) 400 calories, 10 grams of fat
- Cream-filled doughnut (1 doughnut) 310 calories, 21 grams of fat
- Carrot cake with icing (1 average slice) 485 calories, 10-35 gram of fat

Do the math: 500 extra calories per day for 1 week = 1 pound weight gain

As you begin eating healthier, your body may need time to adjust to new amounts and types of foods. Many Herbalife users don't have any problems. They simply notice how much better they feel. But, as with any weight-loss plan, you may encounter an occasional bump in the road. These are some common problems experienced by any dieter and solutions.

"I FEEL WEAK AND TIRED."

Are you properly mixing your Formula 1 Shakes, with the recommended amounts of milk and Performance Protein Powder?

Did you skip a meal to lose weight faster?

SOLUTION:

Eat every meal on time. Don't skip meals or Formula 1 Shakes and get plenty of rest. If you need extra energy, try Total Control™.

"I'M HUNGRY ALL THE TIME."

Are you really hungry or just craving certain foods?

Are you eating the right amount of protein for your body composition?

SOLUTION:

Maintain a regular meal and snack schedule, such as 7 a.m., 11 a.m., 3 p.m. and 7 p.m. You also may need to increase your protein intake by adding Performance Protein Powder to your shakes or try Snack Defense™.

"I HAVE A HEADACHE."

Have you been constipated or stressed?

Are you skipping meals?

Did you stop drinking coffee or caffeine with your new plan?

SOLUTION:

Eat high-fiber fruits and vegetables. (You also may take Herbalife Activated Fiber Powder supplement.) Eat all your meals and get a reasonable amount of exercise. Feel free to enjoy coffee or tea in the amount that you're used to.

"I FEEL NAUSEOUS."

Do you feel sick to your stomach after taking your supplements?

Does the problem occur often?

SOLUTION:

Be sure to take your tablets with your shakes or with your meals, not on an empty stomach. Make sure that you are drinking enough water each day. Herbalife's Herbal Aloe Drink can also help to settle your stomach, and it tastes great.

"I FEEL COLD."

Have you noticed your body temperature decreasesince you stopped overeating?

Are you more sensitive to temperature changes?

SOLUTION:

Increase your body temperature by exercising, drinking warm tea and coffee and dressing in layers.

"I'M NOT REGULAR."

Do you havea change in your digestive functions?

Is the problem constipation or gas?

SOLUTION:

If taking some fiber each day does not solve constipation problems, try Herbalife Activated Fiber Powder and Herbal Aloe Drink. To combat gas, use an over the counter product for that problem.

"I'M NOT LOSING WEIGHT."

Haveyou kept track of all your snacks?

Have your measured your portions correctly?

SOLUTION:

Sometimes people are unaware of all that they eat. Make sure you are using the on line iChange program and keeping your to keep track of everything you consume and pay attention to the size of your portions. Increased awareness will help you stick closely to your weight loss plan.

Exercise for Shape and Health

Regular exercise is vital to the success of your Healthy Living program, and the benefits can change your life.

- Increase your lean muscle mass to burn more calories
- Raise your metabolic rate to burn even more calories
- Maintain your weight loss over the long term
- Improve your cardiovascular health
- Tone your body and increase your flexibility
- Improve your mental outlook

If you are lucky enough to live in an area where there is a fitness center that uses the Quick Gym ROM machine you will get ultimate benefits in the shortest of time. This uses a combination of high intensity aerobic and resistance exercise so you gain the most benefits in the least amount of time.

Exercise is just as important as your eating plan for losing weight and improving your health. Maximize your weight loss progress with a personal fitness plan that includes both aerobic and anaerobic exercise.

AEROBIC EXERCISE

Aerobic exercise involves large muscle movements over a sustained period of time. Running, fast walking and exercise classes are good examples. You breathe harder, your heart beats faster and great things happen.

- More oxygen reaches your body, and oxygen burns fat.
- Your metabolic rate increases, burning more calories.
- You build muscle as you lose fat.
- Your heart and cardiovascular system become much healthier.
- Your mood improves, as exercise relieves feelings of stress and frustration.

Exercise can be fun, once you make it a regular part of your life. Commit to doing some sort of aerobic exercise every day, and you'll be amazed at how much better you look and feel.

Resistance Training

Strength training has many benefits such as increased strength of your muscles, tendons and ligaments. This will reduce your risk for injury and the increased muscle mass will raise your metabolism and make it easier to maintain a healthy body weight.

PERSONALIZE YOUR EXERCISE

Exercise doesn't have to be a struggle, but if you want to be lean and healthy, you've got to work for it. Choose exercise options that give you the benefits that you need and ones that you'll enjoy: organized programs, recreational outlets, sports and gentler lifestyle activities. Select several that are right for you. Then, get moving and stay with it!

Exercise is important to develop your body, but it's just as important to make time to unwind. Meditation and stretching are effective ways to relax your mind and body.

MEDITATION

With a little practice, regular meditation will help lower your blood pressure, body temperature and breathing rate, to give your body a break from the stresses of everyday life.

Take a few moments to try this relaxing meditation exercise.

- Set aside at least five minutes when you won't be interrupted.
- Lie flat on a level surface with a pillow under your head.
- Close your eyes.
- Count to three as you slowly inhale
- Count to four as you slowly exhale.
- Think only about your breathing.

When you feel relaxed, slowly open your eyes and resume normal breath- ing. If you have difficulty keeping your mind on your breathing, focus on a relaxing image or word.

When you can successfully meditate for five minutes, gradually increase your time until reach a full 30-minute session.

Stretching

If meditating is difficult for you, try stretching or yoga. Enroll in a class, or get a book, and do it yourself! Stretching and yoga can reduce stress in your muscles and joints. This is especially valuable if you work long hours at a desk, which builds tension in the muscles of your neck, back, shoulders and chest.

These simple stretches can help.

- Stand up every 30 minutes.
- Rotate your head fully.
- Shrug your shoulders several times.
- Stretch your arms in front of you and move them back and forth.
- Bend your elbows behind you

Dining Out

Tips for Healthy Eating While Dining Out

Even though menu planning and meal selection is best when performed at home, there are still healthy ways to eat when you are dining out. Everyone loves to have a dinner in a wonderful restaurant. You do not have to worry about who will do the dishes and you can avoid the whole cooking process, but restaurant meals tend to be real diet-breakers. Filled with fat, cholesterol and sodium, many restaurant foods taste delicious but offer none of the nutrients that a healthy body requires. Restaurants are renowned for cooking with huge amounts of butter and salt, 2 things that we really want to avoid when it comes to healthy eating.

Tip #1 - Keep It Simple

To avoid eating those foods that are going to knock your diet out of the park, stick to simple choices. If you can find something on the menu that is raw, steamed, grilled, broiled or baked, choose that item. In general, the less preparation that a food requires in order to make it edible, the more nutritious this food is for your body. This means that raw vegetables and fruits come first when you make your appetizer selection. If you can have a small salad as an appetizer, do that first. Pick the raw fruits and vegetables before you choose the meat for your entree. Steamed vegetables retain much of their nutrients as do baked vegetables. Avoiding fried foods is just the beginning when eating in a restaurant. Try to also avoid foods that are pureed because butter or heavy cream is often added to the puree.

Tip #2 - Avoid The Grease

This tip might seem a little over-used, but there is no better way to cut fat from your diet than by avoiding anything that is breaded and deep fried. Many restaurants serve deep fried cheese or vegetables as an appetizer. There is no real nutritional value in a vegetable once it has been covered in butter, egg and breading and doused in oil. If you can eat dinner without choosing any fried items from the menu, you have taken a big step toward healthier living and eating. Oils also hide in places that you probably would not suspect immediately. Remember that pan fried items are generally cooked in oils, as well. So that pan-fried tilapia is not as healthy as you might think. Restaurants are notorious for choosing butter over healthier fats like olive oil because butter tends to be less expansive and of course, tastes delicious.

Tip #3 - Watch Your Portion Sizes

A great way to save money and calories and fat is by eating an early-bird special at a restaurant. These meals are often smaller than the standard portions served for dinner and they come at a much lower price. Portion sizes are one of the worst mistakes that are made in nutrition. Although a small amount of fried chicken or a pat of butter is not terrible for your body, half of a fried chicken is pretty bad. Many restaurants serve huge portions in hopes of giving diners value for their money. Do you really need to eat 1/4 of a chicken at dinner? If the restaurant offers huge portions, divide your meal immediately into 2 smaller meals. Ask your waitress for a "to-go" box and place half of the meal in the box as soon as you receive the plate. This limits the quantity of food that you will eat at that meal without making you feel as if you are missing something.

Tip #4 - Skip The Sugary Drinks

When you order your meal at a restaurant, order water with the meal. Rather than drinking a giant soda that is loaded with sugar and calories, choose water with lemon. If you just cannot live without a soda, only order the smallest size. Many drinks come in such a large size that they will contain 300 calories or more and include 20 tablespoons of sugar. Water is vitally important for your body to function well and most of us do not get enough of it. Have water with your meal and you can splurge on a tiny dessert without the guilt. Water with lemon is flavorful and free.

Tip #5 – Try "Family Style" Ordering

Instead of having each person in your party order a separate appetizer and meal, try a family style order. Pick 2 or 3 appetizers and 2 or 3 entrees and share them between everyone in your party. This gives you a taste of many different menu items without the feeling that you must finish your entire plate of food. Since most restaurants serve huge portions anyway, family style dining is a great way to save money and enjoy the largest variety of food on the menu. Remember that you still need to stick to healthy options, so try an order of broiled fish or chicken and wild rice with appetizers that consist of foods that are not overly processed.

Tip #6 - Skip The Sauce

Even healthy dishes can become incredibly fattening when you put sauce on them. Broiled chicken is delicious, but add that garlic and cream sauce and you have taken all of the "healthy" out of the meal. If a meal requires a special sauce, ask your waiter to serve the sauce on the side. This rule applies to salads and dips as well as for meals. Even the most nutritious item on the menu is not good for you if you soak it in butter and heavy cream. Rather than avoiding sauce altogether, simply order it on the side and dip your fork into the sauce while you eat. You will have all of the flavor without the huge amount of fat and calories.

Restaurant dining is an important part of many of our lives. With hectic lives and busy schedules it is impossible to cook a meal at home every day. Choosing your entrees wisely will give you control over your nutrition and your diet when dining out.

Healthy Living Herbalife Weight Loss Product Suggestions:

Start with the core products:

Formula 1 Healthy meal nutrition shake mix - Treat your body to a healthy, balanced meal in no time! Not only are these shakes easy to make, they're also delicious. With up to 21 essential vitamins and minerals – and in a variety of flavors – weight management never tasted so good! Part of the Herbalife Nutrition.

Formula 2 Multivitamin Complex - A daily multivitamin in tablet form with 21 essential micronutrients, including folic acid, calcium and iron, and antioxidant Vitamins A (as beta-carotene), C and E.

Formula 3 Cell Activator - Formula 3 Cell Activator® supports normal mitochondrial function with alpha-lipoic acid and may help the body's absorption of micronutrients with aloe vera.

Weight Loss Enhancers in beneficial order:

Herbal Tea Concentrate - Herbal Tea Concentrate contains caffeine which jump-starts your metabolism and provides a boost to help you feel revitalized. For optimum experience, mix a a little more than ½ teaspoon with 8 ounces of water. This refreshing, low-calorie tea is available in a variety of flavors.

Total Control – Total Control® tablets contain a proprietary blend of tea extracts and caffeine which quickly stimulates metabolism and provides an energetic and alert feeling.

Cell-U-Loss – Formulated with corn silk, an herb traditionally used to support healthy elimination of water.

Snack Defense – Support your weight-management program with gymnema and chromium in Snack Defense®, which help keep post-meal blood sugar peaks within the normal range.

Thermo-Bond – Thermo-Bond® is formulated with sodium choleate and a fiber blend containing cellulose, apple, acacia, oat and citrus.

Prolessa® Duo – This dual-action formula supports your weight-loss program with two clinically tested ingredients: conjugated linoleic acid and a blend of palm and oat oils.

Personalized Protein Powder - Personalized Protein Powder is a high-quality protein blend that supports your weight-management and fitness goals. Increased protein intake helps you feel fuller longer and maintain your energy level between meals.

Protein Drink Mix – Satisfy your hunger and stay energized with the power of protein! Add Protein Drink Mix to your favorite Formula 1 shake to boost your protein intake to 24 g (without the addition of milk) or mix with water for a nutritious protein snack.

We have many other products to help with your nutritional needs. These can be found at our site at http://herbalnutrition.com/rodstone. And remember join our auto program and you will get 15% off of your products automatically delivered to you every month.